Healing With Iodine

Incorporating Iodine for Healing

By

Baylen Aston

Table of Contents

CHAPTER 1

Introduction

The use of iodine in healing and medicine has a storied history dating back centuries, encompassing a spectrum of traditional remedies and modern medical applications. Iodine, a chemical element denoted by the symbol 'I' in the periodic table, holds a pivotal role in maintaining human health.

1.1 Background and Significance

Background:

Iodine, a non-metallic trace element, is an indispensable component of the human diet, and its physiological importance cannot be overstated. It plays a fundamental role in the functioning of the thyroid gland, a vital organ responsible for regulating metabolic processes through the production of thyroid hormones. Iodine, in the form of iodide ions (I-), is absorbed through dietary intake, predominantly from iodized salt, seafood, and certain dairy products.

The historical context of iodine's significance in human health is rich and diverse. Ancient civilizations, notably the Egyptians and Greeks, recognized its therapeutic properties, utilizing iodine-rich seaweed and marine-derived compounds in various medicinal concoctions. However, it was not until the 19th century that iodine's role in healing became more systematically explored and understood. The development of iodine-based antiseptics by pioneering physicians such as Ignaz Semmelweis and Joseph Lister revolutionized surgical practices, drastically reducing postoperative infections and mortality rates.

Significance:

The significance of studying iodine's healing properties extends beyond historical curiosity. In contemporary healthcare, iodine continues to be an essential tool, particularly in the realms of wound care, antiseptic procedures, and thyroid management. Its contributions to infection control, tissue repair, and thyroid function have positioned iodine as a critical agent in modern medicine.

Moreover, iodine's significance is amplified by the global issue of iodine deficiency. Despite substantial progress in addressing this problem through iodized salt programs, regions still experience deficiencies that lead to widespread health concerns, including goiter, cognitive impairments, and developmental issues, especially in pregnant women and infants. Understanding the role of iodine in healing can provide insights into strategies for combatting these deficiencies and their associated health consequences.

1.2 Importance of Iodine for Healing

Iodine is an essential trace element that plays a crucial role in maintaining the health of the thyroid gland and supporting overall bodily functions. While iodine does have some roles in wound healing, its importance in healing isn't as pronounced as its role in thyroid function and overall health.

1. **Thyroid Function**: Iodine is a fundamental component of thyroid hormones, such as thyroxine (T4) and triiodothyronine (T3). These hormones are vital for regulating metabolism, energy production, and overall bodily functions.

2. **Wound Healing**: Iodine has antiseptic properties that help prevent infections in wounds and cuts. It can be used topically to disinfect wounds, reducing the risk of bacterial growth and promoting faster healing.

3. **Antibacterial Agent**: Iodine has broad-spectrum antibacterial properties, making

it effective against various types of bacteria, fungi, and even some viruses. It can be used to disinfect surfaces and prevent infection in medical settings.

4. **Anti-Inflammatory**: Iodine's anti-inflammatory properties can help reduce swelling and inflammation, which are common responses to injuries or infections.

5. **Immune System Support**: Iodine supports the immune system by aiding in the production of white blood cells, which are essential for fighting off infections and promoting healing.

6. **Cell Regeneration**: Iodine is necessary for cellular

regeneration and repair. It promotes the growth and maintenance of healthy cells, which is crucial for tissue healing and recovery.

7. **Collagen Synthesis**: Iodine is involved in the synthesis of collagen, a protein that provides structural support to skin, blood vessels, tendons, and other connective tissues. Collagen is essential for wound healing and tissue repair.

8. **Hormone Balance**: Proper iodine levels contribute to hormone balance, which is important for various bodily processes, including growth, development, and reproductive health.

9. **Detoxification**: Iodine supports the body's detoxification processes, helping to remove harmful substances and toxins from the body. This can contribute to a healthier environment for healing.

10. **Bone Health**: Adequate iodine levels are important for maintaining bone health. Iodine deficiency can lead to decreased bone mineral density, which may affect the healing of bone injuries.

It's important to note that while iodine is essential for healing, both deficiency and excess can have negative effects on the body. Mild iodine deficiency can impair the healing process, while excessive iodine intake can lead to thyroid dysfunction and other health issues.

Therefore, it's recommended to maintain a balanced and appropriate level of iodine intake, either through dietary sources (such as iodized salt, seafood, and dairy products) or under medical supervision when using iodine-based treatments.

CHAPTER 2

Iodine: An Essential Element

Iodine is a remarkable chemical element that plays a pivotal role in maintaining human health. This section will delve into the various aspects of iodine's importance, starting with its presence in the human body, its dietary sources, and the critical issue of iodine deficiency and its far-reaching health implications.

2.1 Iodine in the Human Body

Iodine is primarily found in the thyroid gland, an essential organ situated in the neck. This gland is responsible for the synthesis and secretion of thyroid hormones, chiefly thyroxine (T4) and triiodothyronine (T3). These hormones are integral to regulating the body's metabolic processes, including energy production, temperature regulation, and protein synthesis.

The unique feature of thyroid hormones is that they contain iodine atoms. T4, for instance, contains four iodine atoms, while T3 contains three. These hormones are released into the bloodstream in precise quantities to orchestrate metabolism in virtually every cell of the body. The availability of iodine directly influences the thyroid's ability to produce these hormones, making iodine an essential element for overall health.

2.2 Dietary Sources of Iodine

The human body cannot synthesize iodine on its own, making dietary intake crucial for maintaining adequate iodine levels. While iodine can be found in various foods, certain sources are particularly rich in this element. The primary dietary sources of iodine include:

- **Iodized Salt:** One of the most effective public health interventions, iodized salt contains added iodine, ensuring a reliable and accessible source of this essential element in many diets worldwide.

- **Seafood:** Seafood, especially fish and shellfish, is abundant in iodine due to the ocean's iodine-rich environment. Seaweeds, such as kelp and nori, are particularly iodine-dense and are commonly used in Asian cuisines.

- **Dairy Products:** Milk and dairy products, like cheese and yogurt, are good sources of iodine, as dairy animals typically consume iodine-rich feed.

- **Eggs:** Eggs can also contribute to iodine intake, albeit in smaller amounts compared to seafood and dairy.

- **Iodine Supplements:** In regions where, natural dietary sources are scarce, iodine supplements or iodine-fortified foods may be recommended to prevent deficiency.

2.3 Iodine Deficiency and Health Implications

Iodine deficiency is a global health concern with significant health implications, particularly in regions where dietary iodine sources are limited. When the body lacks sufficient iodine to produce thyroid hormones, several health problems can arise:

- **Goiter:** A visibly enlarged thyroid gland, known as a goiter, is a classic sign of iodine deficiency. It occurs as the thyroid gland attempts to compensate for the lack of iodine by enlarging in a futile effort to produce more hormones.

- **Hypothyroidism:** Iodine deficiency can lead to an underactive thyroid, a condition known as hypothyroidism. Symptoms may include fatigue, weight gain, cold intolerance, and cognitive impairments.

- **Developmental Issues:** Iodine deficiency during pregnancy and infancy can result in severe developmental issues, including intellectual disabilities, stunted growth, and developmental delays in children.

- **Thyroid Disorders:** Inadequate iodine intake can also contribute to various thyroid disorders, including thyroid nodules and autoimmune conditions like Hashimoto's thyroiditis.

Understanding the importance of iodine in the human body and recognizing the consequences of iodine deficiency underscores the critical role of this element in maintaining overall health. In subsequent sections, we will explore how iodine's healing properties extend to both traditional and modern medical practices, further highlighting its significance in the field of medicine and healthcare.

CHAPTER 3

Historical Uses of Iodine in Healing

The historical uses of iodine in healing reveal a fascinating journey that spans centuries, showcasing the evolution from ancient remedies and practices to its emergence as a valuable tool in modern medicine.

3.1 Ancient Remedies and Practices

Ancient Egypt and Greece:

The use of iodine-rich substances in healing dates back to ancient civilizations, most notably in Egypt and Greece. In Egypt, iodine-containing seaweed and algae were used as part of various medicinal concoctions. The Egyptians recognized the therapeutic potential of these marine-derived substances, employing them to treat wounds and skin ailments.

Similarly, in ancient Greece, the renowned physician Hippocrates noted the healing properties of iodine-rich seaweed. Greek physicians incorporated these marine resources into treatments for thyroid-related conditions and goiter, although they lacked the scientific understanding of iodine's specific role.

Traditional Asian Medicine:

In traditional Asian medicine, particularly in countries like Japan and China, seaweed-based remedies were used for centuries. Seaweeds rich in iodine were administered to address thyroid-related disorders and promote overall health. These practices laid the foundation for later scientific investigations into iodine's healing potential.

3.2 Iodine's Emergence in Modern Medicine

19th Century Breakthroughs:

The 19th century marked a pivotal era for iodine's emergence in modern medicine. Several key developments during this period propelled iodine into the forefront of medical practice:

- **Iodine-Based Antiseptics:** Ignaz Semmelweis and later Joseph Lister revolutionized surgical practices by introducing iodine-based antiseptics. Semmelweis's pioneering work on handwashing with iodine solutions significantly reduced postoperative infections, demonstrating the critical role of hand hygiene in healthcare settings. Lister, building on Semmelweis's findings, developed carbolic acid, a derivative of iodine, as an antiseptic for surgical instruments and wound care. These breakthroughs dramatically improved patient outcomes and paved the way for modern aseptic techniques.

- **Treatment of Goiter:** Physicians in the 19th century began to experiment with iodine as a treatment for goiter, a condition characterized by an enlarged thyroid gland. The administration of iodine supplements and iodine-rich substances was found to shrink goiters, providing tangible evidence of iodine's efficacy in thyroid-related disorders.

- **Iodine Tincture:** Iodine tincture, a solution of iodine and potassium iodide, was developed as a topical antiseptic. It became a staple in first-aid kits and was widely used for disinfecting wounds, a practice that continued well into the 20th century.

- **Iodine for Thyroid Health:** As understanding of thyroid function deepened, iodine's importance in thyroid health became increasingly evident. Iodine supplementation and the development of iodized salt, introduced in the early 20th century, played a pivotal role in mitigating iodine deficiency and associated thyroid disorders.

Iodine's journey from ancient remedies to its integral role in modern medicine exemplifies the dynamic relationship between traditional knowledge and scientific progress. Today, iodine remains a fundamental element in healthcare, with applications extending beyond antiseptic and thyroid-related treatments to encompass diverse fields, such as wound care, surgical procedures, and emerging medical technologies. In the subsequent sections, we will delve further into the mechanisms and benefits of healing with iodine, shedding light on its multifaceted contributions to the world of medicine.

CHAPTER 4

Healing with Iodine: Mechanisms and Benefits

Iodine's remarkable healing properties are rooted in its versatile mechanisms and numerous benefits, which extend to both its role as an antiseptic and its contributions to wound healing.

4.1 Antiseptic Properties of Iodine

Iodine's efficacy as an antiseptic is a well-established aspect of its healing potential. Its antiseptic properties are harnessed in various forms, such as iodine tincture and povidone-iodine solutions. Here are the key mechanisms and benefits of iodine as an antiseptic:

- **Microbial Inhibition:** Iodine is highly effective at killing or inhibiting the growth of a broad spectrum of microorganisms, including bacteria, viruses, fungi, and even some parasites. This makes it an invaluable tool for disinfecting wounds, surgical sites, and medical equipment.

- **Oxidative Stress:** Iodine exerts its antimicrobial effects by inducing oxidative stress in microorganisms. It disrupts their cell membranes, proteins, and nucleic acids, leading to cell death. This oxidative action is rapid and effective against both surface pathogens and those that may be deeper within tissues.

- **Low Resistance:** Microorganisms have a low resistance to iodine, which reduces the likelihood of developing iodine-resistant strains. This is in contrast to some other antimicrobial agents, where resistance can emerge more readily.

- **Non-Toxicity to Human Cells:** Iodine's antiseptic properties are selectively toxic to microorganisms, sparing human cells from harm when used appropriately. This selectivity is a crucial advantage in medical applications.

- **Wound Infection Prevention:** Iodine-based antiseptics are widely used to prevent wound infections, particularly in surgical settings. They are applied to the skin before surgery to reduce the risk of introducing harmful microorganisms into the body.

4.2 Iodine's Role in Wound Healing

Iodine's contributions to wound healing extend beyond its antiseptic properties, encompassing several mechanisms that promote the recovery of injured tissues:

- **Infection Control:** As an antiseptic, iodine helps prevent infections in wounds, which is essential for the proper healing process. Infections can delay healing and lead to complications.

- **Reduction of Inflammation:** Iodine can help modulate the inflammatory response in wounds. While inflammation is a natural part of the healing process, excessive inflammation can hinder healing. Iodine may help regulate this response.

- **Collagen Production:** Iodine is involved in the synthesis of collagen, a structural protein crucial for wound repair. Adequate collagen formation is necessary for the strength and integrity of healed tissues.

- **Angiogenesis:** Iodine has been shown to stimulate the formation of new blood vessels, a process known as angiogenesis. Improved blood supply to the wound site facilitates the delivery of oxygen and nutrients, promoting tissue regeneration.

- **Epithelialization:** Iodine supports the migration and proliferation of epithelial cells, which are responsible for covering the wound with a protective layer of skin. This process, called epithelialization, is a key step in wound closure.

- **Reduction of Scar Tissue:** Some studies suggest that iodine may help reduce the formation of excessive scar tissue (keloids and hypertrophic scars) by promoting more controlled collagen deposition.

- **Pain Relief:** Iodine may have analgesic (pain-relieving) properties, which can enhance the comfort of individuals during the healing process.

The combined action of iodine as an antiseptic and its role in wound healing makes it a valuable asset in various healthcare settings, from surgical theaters to first aid. Understanding these mechanisms and benefits underscores iodine's versatility and effectiveness in promoting the healing of wounds and preventing infections, ultimately contributing to better patient outcomes.

4.3 Iodine's Impact on Thyroid Health

Iodine plays a central role in thyroid health, and its availability is crucial for the proper functioning of this vital endocrine gland. Here, we delve into how iodine influences thyroid health, the consequences of deficiency, and the broader implications for overall well-being.

4.3.1 Thyroid Hormone Synthesis

The thyroid gland is responsible for producing thyroid hormones, primarily thyroxine (T4) and triiodothyronine (T3). These hormones are essential for regulating metabolic processes throughout the body. Iodine is a fundamental component of these thyroid hormones, accounting for the "triiodo" in T3 and the "tetraiodo" in T4. The synthesis of these hormones is a complex process that relies on the availability of iodine in the body.

1. **Iodine Uptake:** The thyroid gland actively takes up iodine from the bloodstream using a specialized transporter called the sodium-iodine symporter (NIS). This process is regulated by the thyroid-

stimulating hormone (TSH) released by the pituitary gland.

2. **Thyroglobulin Production:** Iodine is incorporated into thyroglobulin, a protein synthesized by the thyroid gland. Thyroglobulin acts as a scaffold for thyroid hormone production.

3. **Hormone Synthesis:** Iodine atoms are added to thyroglobulin to form T3 and T4 molecules. T4 is the major thyroid hormone produced by the thyroid, while T3 is the more biologically active form.

4. **Hormone Release:** When needed, the thyroid gland releases T3 and T4 into the bloodstream, where they travel to target tissues and organs. These hormones play a critical role in regulating

metabolism, body temperature, heart rate, and energy production.

4.3.2 Iodine Deficiency and Thyroid Disorders

Iodine deficiency can have profound implications for thyroid health:

1. **Goiter:** A common consequence of iodine deficiency is the development of a goiter, which is an enlarged thyroid gland. In an effort to obtain more iodine, the thyroid gland enlarges, resulting in a visibly swollen neck. This is a compensatory mechanism to increase iodine uptake and hormone production.

2. **Hypothyroidism:** Prolonged iodine deficiency can lead to hypothyroidism, a condition characterized by an underactive thyroid gland. In hypothyroidism,

insufficient thyroid hormone production can cause symptoms such as fatigue, weight gain, cold intolerance, and cognitive impairments.

3. **Thyroid Autoimmune Diseases:** Iodine deficiency may contribute to autoimmune thyroid diseases, such as Hashimoto's thyroiditis, where the immune system mistakenly attacks the thyroid gland. These conditions can lead to chronic inflammation and further impair thyroid function.

4. **Pregnancy and Developmental Issues:** Iodine deficiency during pregnancy and infancy can have severe consequences, including intellectual disabilities in children (cretinism), developmental delays, and impaired growth.

4.3.3 Iodine Supplementation and Health Considerations

While iodine deficiency is a serious concern, excessive iodine intake can also have adverse effects on thyroid health. Therefore, it is essential to strike a balance between ensuring adequate iodine intake and avoiding excessive exposure.

1. **Iodized Salt:** In many countries, iodized salt is a crucial source of iodine. It provides a consistent and controlled dose of iodine, making it an effective means of preventing deficiency.

2. **Supplementation:** In regions with persistent iodine deficiency, iodine supplements or iodine-fortified foods may be recommended under

medical supervision to address the deficiency.

3. **Balanced Intake:** Maintaining a balanced iodine intake is crucial. Excessive iodine from supplements or naturally iodine-rich foods (e.g., seaweed) can lead to thyroid dysfunction, including hyperthyroidism.

Iodine's impact on thyroid health is profound and multifaceted. It is indispensable for the synthesis of thyroid hormones, which regulate crucial metabolic functions in the body. Understanding the role of iodine in thyroid health underscores its critical importance and emphasizes the need for balanced iodine intake to prevent both deficiency-related and excess-related thyroid disorders.

CHAPTER 5

Iodine Applications in Medical Settings

Iodine has found diverse applications in medical settings, ranging from its use as a topical antiseptic to more specialized applications in surgical procedures and pharmaceuticals. In this section, we will explore the role of iodine in medical disinfection and its use in topical solutions.

5.1 Topical Iodine Solutions and Disinfection

Iodine's antiseptic properties make it a valuable tool in medical disinfection, especially for skin and mucous membrane preparations. Here, we focus on its use in topical iodine solutions and its role in maintaining aseptic conditions in various healthcare contexts:

Pre-Surgical Skin Preparation: Before surgical procedures, it is crucial to disinfect the patient's skin to reduce the risk of postoperative infections. Topical iodine solutions, such as povidone-iodine (commonly known as Betadine), are commonly used for this purpose. These solutions are applied to the surgical site to eliminate or significantly reduce the microbial load on the skin, creating a sterile field for the operation.

Wound Care: Iodine-based solutions are employed for wound care, particularly in the management of contaminated or infected wounds. The antiseptic properties of iodine help to cleanse wounds by killing or inhibiting the growth of bacteria and other pathogens. This promotes a healthier wound environment conducive to healing.

Emergency and First Aid: Iodine solutions are valuable in emergency and first aid situations. They can be used to disinfect minor cuts, abrasions, and burns, reducing the risk of infection. Iodine's broad-spectrum antimicrobial action makes it an effective choice for preventing the introduction of pathogens into wounds.

Mucous Membrane Disinfection: In medical and dental procedures involving mucous membranes, iodine-based solutions can be used to disinfect the oral and nasal cavities, as well as the genital and rectal areas. This is crucial for reducing the risk of infection during invasive procedures and examinations.

Intravenous Site Preparation: Iodine-based solutions are used to prepare the skin at intravenous (IV) catheter insertion sites. This helps maintain a sterile environment around the catheter, minimizing the chances of catheter-related infections.

Nail and Skin Infections: Topical iodine solutions are sometimes prescribed for the treatment of fungal nail infections (onychomycosis) and certain skin infections, as they can penetrate tissues to target the underlying pathogens.

Patient Decolonization: In some cases, healthcare providers may use iodine-based solutions to decolonize patients who are carriers of antibiotic-resistant bacteria like MRSA

(Methicillin-resistant Staphylococcus aureus) to prevent the spread of infections within healthcare facilities.

It's important to note that while iodine-based antiseptics are highly effective, they must be used with care and in accordance with established protocols. Povidone-iodine, for instance, should not be used on individuals with iodine allergies, and healthcare professionals should consider factors such as iodine sensitivity and the potential for skin irritation when selecting antiseptics.

Iodine's use in medical disinfection, particularly in the form of topical solutions, is a critical component of infection control in healthcare settings. Its broad-spectrum antimicrobial properties make it a valuable tool for creating and maintaining aseptic conditions, whether in surgical theaters, wound care, or emergency situations.

5.2 Iodine-Based Pharmaceuticals

Iodine-based pharmaceuticals encompass a wide range of medicinal products and treatments that utilize the unique properties of iodine for therapeutic purposes. These pharmaceuticals have applications across various medical disciplines, and their effectiveness stems from iodine's antimicrobial, antiseptic, and contrast-enhancing properties. Here, we explore some of the key iodine-based pharmaceuticals and their medical applications:

1. **Iodine-Containing Contrast Agents:**

- **Iodine-based contrast agents** are commonly used in medical imaging procedures such as computed tomography (CT) scans and angiography. These agents enhance the visibility of blood vessels, organs, and tissues in radiographic images, allowing healthcare providers to obtain clearer and more detailed diagnostic information.

- **Iodine-based contrast agents** are either administered orally or injected intravenously. Their ability to absorb X-rays makes them indispensable tools in diagnostic radiology, helping to visualize structures that would otherwise be difficult to discern.

2. Iodine-Containing Radiopharmaceuticals:

- **Iodine-131 (I-131)** is used in nuclear medicine for diagnostic and therapeutic purposes. It emits beta particles and gamma rays, making it suitable for imaging and treatment of thyroid disorders and certain types of cancer. I-131 is commonly employed in radioactive iodine therapy for thyroid cancer and hyperthyroidism.

3. **Topical Antiseptics:**

- **Povidone-iodine**, often known by its brand name Betadine, is a widely used iodine-based antiseptic. It is used in various topical formulations, including solutions, ointments, and gels. Povidone-iodine is utilized for disinfecting skin and mucous membranes before surgical procedures and as a general antiseptic for wound care. It helps prevent infections and supports wound healing.

4. Iodine Supplements:

- **Iodine supplements** are available in various forms, including potassium iodide and sodium iodide. They are used to treat iodine deficiency, which can lead to thyroid disorders and developmental issues. Iodine supplements are prescribed under medical supervision to ensure adequate intake without excessive exposure.

5. Iodine-Based Pharmaceuticals in Dermatology:

- **Iodine-based pharmaceuticals** are sometimes used in dermatology for the treatment of skin conditions. Iodine tincture, for instance, may be employed to treat skin infections, fungal nail infections, and certain types of dermatitis.

6. Iodine-Based Wound Dressings:

- **Iodine-based wound dressings** incorporate iodine into wound care products. These dressings release iodine gradually, creating an antimicrobial environment in the wound while promoting healing. They are used for chronic and infected wounds.

7. Iodine-Based Radioprotectants:

- **Potassium iodide** can serve as a radioprotectant in nuclear emergencies. When administered before or shortly after exposure to radioactive iodine, it saturates the thyroid gland with non-radioactive iodine, reducing the uptake of radioactive iodine and the risk of thyroid cancer.

It's important to note that while iodine-based pharmaceuticals offer significant therapeutic benefits, they should be used under the guidance of healthcare professionals. Iodine, like any medication, can have side effects and contraindications, and its use should be tailored to individual patient needs and medical conditions.

Iodine-based pharmaceuticals encompass a diverse array of medical interventions that leverage iodine's properties for diagnostic, therapeutic, and preventive purposes. These pharmaceuticals play a vital role in modern medicine, aiding in diagnostics, treatments, and maintaining aseptic conditions for surgical procedures.

5.3 Iodine and Surgical Procedures

Iodine plays a crucial role in maintaining aseptic conditions during surgical procedures. Its antimicrobial properties make it an invaluable tool for preventing surgical site infections and ensuring patient safety. Here, we explore the use of iodine in surgical settings and its various applications:

1. Preoperative Skin Preparation:

- **Skin Disinfection:** One of the primary applications of iodine in surgery is preoperative skin preparation. Before surgical procedures, it is essential to disinfect the patient's skin in the operative area to reduce the risk of postoperative infections.

- **Iodine-Based Solutions:** Iodine-based solutions, such as povidone-iodine (commonly known as Betadine), are commonly used for this purpose. These solutions are applied to the patient's skin in the surgical field. They help eliminate or significantly reduce the microbial load on the skin, creating a sterile environment for the operation.

- **Hair Removal:** Iodine-based solutions can also be used to remove hair from the surgical site, ensuring a clean surface for incisions and reducing the risk of contamination.

2. Hand Hygiene:

- **Surgeon and Staff Hand Hygiene:** Maintaining proper hand hygiene among surgical personnel is crucial to prevent the introduction of pathogens into the surgical site. Iodine-based handwash solutions or iodine-containing surgical scrub brushes are used by surgeons and staff to disinfect their hands before surgery.

3. Mucous Membrane Disinfection:

- **Mucous Membrane Disinfection:** In surgical procedures involving mucous membranes, such as oral, nasal, genital, or rectal surgeries, iodine-based solutions can be used to disinfect these areas. This is vital for reducing the risk of infection during invasive procedures and examinations.

4. Instrument and Equipment Sterilization:

- **Instrument Sterilization:** Iodine-based solutions can be used to sterilize surgical instruments and equipment. This ensures that all tools used during surgery are free from contaminants that could potentially cause infections.

5. Vaginal Antiseptics:

- **Vaginal Antiseptics:** In obstetrics and gynecology, iodine-based solutions may be used as vaginal antiseptics before certain procedures or childbirth. This helps reduce the risk of maternal and neonatal infections.

6. Antiseptic Drapes:

- **Antiseptic Drapes:** Specialized iodine-impregnated surgical drapes are available. These drapes are placed over the patient, creating a sterile barrier around the surgical site. They provide continuous antimicrobial protection during the procedure.

7. Iodine Sutures:

- **Iodine Sutures:** Some surgical sutures are coated with iodine to provide continuous antimicrobial action at the incision site. This can help reduce the risk of postoperative infections.

It's important to emphasize that while iodine is highly effective in preventing surgical site infections, its use should be in accordance with established protocols and under the supervision of healthcare professionals. Iodine allergies or sensitivities should also be considered when using iodine-based products in surgical settings.

Iodine's role in surgical procedures is indispensable for maintaining aseptic conditions, preventing infections, and ensuring patient safety. Its broad-spectrum antimicrobial properties make it a vital component of modern surgical practices, contributing to successful outcomes and reducing the risk of postoperative complications.

CHAPTER 6

Controversies and Considerations

Iodine usage, whether for medical or dietary purposes, is not without controversies and potential side effects. While iodine is essential for overall health, its intake must be carefully monitored to avoid adverse outcomes. In this section, we explore some of the potential side effects and considerations associated with iodine usage:

6.1 Potential Side Effects of Iodine Usage

1. **Iodine Allergy:** Some individuals may be allergic to iodine. Allergic reactions can range from mild skin irritation to more severe symptoms, such as difficulty breathing or anaphylaxis. Healthcare providers must be aware of a patient's iodine allergy history when using iodine-based products.

2. **Thyroid Dysfunction:** Excessive iodine intake can disrupt thyroid function, leading to thyroid disorders. Both iodine deficiency and iodine excess can result in hypothyroidism or hyperthyroidism, which have a range of symptoms and health implications.

3. **Hyperthyroidism:** High doses of iodine, such as those found in certain supplements or radiographic contrast agents, can trigger or worsen hyperthyroidism in susceptible individuals. Symptoms may include rapid heart rate, weight loss, nervousness, and tremors.

4. **Thyroid Autoimmunity:** Excessive iodine intake has been associated with an increased risk of autoimmune thyroid diseases, such as Hashimoto's thyroiditis and Graves' disease, where the immune system attacks the thyroid gland.

5. **Thyroiditis:** Iodine exposure, particularly in the form of iodinated contrast media, can lead to iodine-induced thyroiditis, a transient inflammation of the

thyroid gland. This condition can cause pain, swelling, and temporary thyroid dysfunction.

6. **GI Disturbances:** High doses of iodine can lead to gastrointestinal disturbances, including nausea, vomiting, and diarrhea.

7. **Skin Irritation:** Topical iodine-based products, if used excessively or on sensitive skin, can cause skin irritation, redness, or dermatitis.

8. **Kidney Function:** Iodine-containing contrast agents can put additional strain on the kidneys, particularly in individuals with preexisting kidney issues.

9. **Pregnancy and Lactation:** Excessive iodine intake during pregnancy can have adverse effects on fetal thyroid development. It's crucial for

pregnant and breastfeeding individuals to maintain an appropriate but not excessive iodine intake to support their own health and their baby's development.

10. **Drug Interactions:** Iodine supplements or contrast agents can interact with certain medications, affecting their absorption or metabolism. Healthcare providers should be aware of potential drug interactions when prescribing iodine-containing products.

11. **Iodine-Induced Acne:** In rare cases, high doses of iodine, such as those found in iodine supplements or kelp-based dietary supplements, have been associated with the development or exacerbation of acne.

It's important to note that iodine requirements can vary greatly among individuals, and the tolerable upper intake levels established by health authorities should be considered to prevent excess iodine intake. Healthcare providers play a critical role in assessing iodine status, addressing deficiencies, and monitoring iodine supplementation to ensure optimal health outcomes.

While iodine is essential for health, its usage should be approached with caution. The potential side effects and considerations associated with iodine underscore the importance of balanced iodine intake, tailored to individual needs and medical conditions, and supervised by healthcare professionals when necessary.

6.2 Debates Surrounding Iodine Supplementation

Iodine supplementation is a topic of ongoing debate and consideration in the field of nutrition and healthcare. While iodine is crucial for overall health, the question of who should receive supplementation, in what form, and at what dosage remains complex. Here, we delve into the debates and considerations surrounding iodine supplementation:

6.2.1 Universal vs. Targeted Supplementation

Universal Supplementation:

- **Pros:** Some argue for universal iodine supplementation, particularly through iodized salt, to ensure that entire populations receive an adequate intake. Universal supplementation has been successful in many regions, effectively addressing iodine deficiency disorders (IDDs).

- **Cons:** Critics of universal supplementation argue that it can lead to excess iodine intake in some individuals, potentially causing thyroid dysfunction. They suggest that a one-size-fits-all approach may not be suitable for all populations, especially in regions where iodine deficiency is not a widespread issue.

Targeted Supplementation:

- **Pros:** Targeted supplementation aims to identify and provide iodine supplementation only to individuals or populations at risk of deficiency. This approach prevents excessive iodine intake in those who do not require it.

- **Cons:** Critics of targeted supplementation argue that it can be logistically challenging to identify and reach all individuals at risk, particularly in remote or underserved regions. There is a risk of missing vulnerable populations.

6.2.2 Iodized Salt vs. Supplements

Iodized Salt:

- **Pros:** Iodized salt is a cost-effective and easily accessible source of iodine. It has been successfully used to address iodine deficiency in many countries. It integrates into existing dietary habits and does not require behavior change.

- **Cons:** Critics argue that iodized salt may not provide precise control over iodine intake, as it depends on individuals' salt consumption. In regions where reducing salt intake is a public health priority, iodized salt may not be the preferred method.

Iodine Supplements:

- **Pros:** Iodine supplements offer precise control over iodine dosage, making it suitable for targeted supplementation. They are valuable in situations where iodized salt is not practical or accepted.

- **Cons:** Critics are concerned about the potential for

excessive iodine intake when supplements are used without medical guidance. The risk of thyroid dysfunction is higher with supplements, especially at high doses.

6.2.3 Monitoring and Surveillance

- **Pros:** Effective monitoring and surveillance systems help identify populations at risk of iodine deficiency and assess the impact of iodine supplementation programs. This information can inform decisions about the necessity and type of supplementation.

- **Cons:** Critics argue that monitoring systems can be costly and logistically challenging to implement, particularly in low-resource settings. Inadequate monitoring can lead to a lack of accurate data on iodine status.

6.2.4 Balancing Deficiency and Excess

- **Pros:** Striking the right balance between addressing iodine deficiency and avoiding iodine excess is crucial. This requires careful consideration of dietary habits, cultural factors, and regional iodine status.

- **Cons:** Critics contend that achieving this balance can be challenging, particularly when addressing varying iodine needs within diverse populations. Some individuals may have higher requirements due to genetics or medical conditions.

Iodine supplementation debates revolve around finding the most effective and safe ways to address iodine deficiency while minimizing the risk of excessive iodine intake and associated health issues. The choice between universal or targeted supplementation, the selection of iodized salt or supplements, and the establishment of robust monitoring systems require careful consideration of local contexts and healthcare infrastructure. Decisions regarding iodine supplementation should ideally be evidence-based and tailored to the specific needs of each population.

6.3 Balancing Iodine Intake for Optimal Health

Achieving and maintaining balanced iodine intake is essential for optimal health. Iodine is a trace element that plays a crucial role in various bodily functions, including thyroid function, cognitive development, and immune health. However, both deficiency and excess iodine intake can have adverse health effects. Here, we explore how to balance iodine intake for overall well-being:

1. Dietary Sources of Iodine:

- **Iodized Salt:** In many countries, iodized table salt is a primary dietary source of iodine. Using iodized salt in cooking and meal preparation can help ensure adequate iodine intake.

- **Seafood:** Seafood, such as fish and seaweed, is naturally rich in iodine. Incorporating seafood into your diet can provide a natural source of iodine.

- **Dairy Products:** Dairy products, including milk, cheese, and yogurt, contain iodine, as it is present in cow feed and iodine-containing sanitizing agents used in the dairy industry.

- **Eggs:** Eggs can be a source of iodine, as the nutrient is present in chicken feed.

- **Fruits and Vegetables:** Some fruits and vegetables contain iodine, although the iodine content can vary based on soil iodine levels.

2. Use Iodized Salt Sparingly:

- While iodized salt is an effective way to prevent iodine deficiency, it's essential not to overuse salt, as excessive salt intake can have adverse effects on blood pressure and cardiovascular health. Use iodized salt in moderation.

3. Be Mindful of Processed Foods:

- Many processed foods, such as canned soups and processed meats, contain added salt. These sources of salt may or may not be iodized, so it's important to read food labels and choose products with iodized salt when possible.

4. Balance Iodine-Rich and Iodine-Poor Foods:

- Achieving balance in your diet is key. While some foods are naturally rich in iodine, others are iodine-poor. A well-rounded diet that includes a variety of foods can help maintain a balanced iodine intake.

5. Consider Dietary Preferences and Restrictions:

- Vegetarians and vegans may have different iodine sources than those who consume animal products. Plant-based sources of iodine include iodized salt, seaweed, and iodine-fortified foods.

6. Be Aware of Iodine Supplements:

- Iodine supplements should be used under medical supervision and only when prescribed by a healthcare provider. Self-administering iodine supplements can lead to excessive iodine intake and thyroid dysfunction.

7. Monitor Iodine Status:

- In regions with a history of iodine deficiency or excess, healthcare providers may monitor iodine status through blood or urine tests. These tests can help determine whether iodine supplementation is necessary or if iodine intake needs to be reduced.

8. Consider Individual Needs:

- Individual iodine requirements can vary based on factors like age, sex, life stage (e.g., pregnancy), genetics, and underlying health conditions. Consult with a healthcare provider or registered dietitian to assess your specific iodine needs.

9. Maintain a Healthy Lifestyle:

- Eating a balanced diet, engaging in regular physical activity, and avoiding excessive alcohol and tobacco use are essential components of overall health and can support proper thyroid function and iodine utilization.

Striking the right balance in iodine intake is essential for optimal health. Whether you obtain iodine from dietary sources, iodized salt, or supplements, it's important to be mindful of your individual needs and to avoid both iodine deficiency and excess. A balanced and varied diet, along with awareness of dietary choices and preferences, is key to maintaining iodine intake at appropriate levels for overall well-being. Consulting with healthcare professionals can provide valuable guidance on iodine intake tailored to your specific circumstances.

CHAPTER 7

Research and Scientific Evidence

7.1 Studies on Iodine's Antimicrobial Properties

Iodine's antimicrobial properties have been the subject of extensive research and scientific investigation. These studies have explored the effectiveness of iodine in killing or inhibiting the growth of various microorganisms, including bacteria, viruses, and fungi. Here are some key findings and examples of research on iodine's antimicrobial properties:

1. Antiseptic Action:

- **Povidone-Iodine (Betadine):**
  Povidone-iodine is a widely used
  iodine-based antiseptic. Numerous
  studies have demonstrated its
  effectiveness in reducing bacterial
  load on the skin, mucous
  membranes, and wounds. For
  example, a study published in the
  Journal of Hospital Infection in
  2018 found that povidone-iodine
  was highly effective in reducing
  microbial contamination in
  surgical site preparations.

- **Mouthwash and Oral
  Antiseptics:** Iodine-based
  mouthwashes and oral antiseptics
  have been studied for their ability
  to reduce oral bacteria, including
  those associated with dental plaque
  and gingivitis.

2. Wound Care:

- **Iodine in Wound Dressings:**
  Some wound dressings incorporate
  iodine to create an antimicrobial
  environment in the wound. A
  study published in the
  International Wound Journal in
  2018 examined the use of iodine-
  releasing dressings in chronic
  wounds and found that they could
  help reduce bacterial load and
  promote wound healing.

3. Ophthalmology:

- **Iodine in Ophthalmic Solutions:**
  Iodine-based ophthalmic solutions
  have been used to disinfect the eye
  and prevent eye infections.
  Research has shown their efficacy
  in reducing the risk of
  postoperative eye infections after
  procedures like cataract surgery.

4. Respiratory Infections:

- **Iodine Vapor Inhalation:** Some research has explored the use of iodine vapor inhalation for respiratory infections. A study published in the Journal of Antimicrobial Chemotherapy in 2017 investigated the antimicrobial activity of iodine vapor against airborne bacteria, including drug-resistant strains.

5. Water Purification:

- **Iodine for Water Disinfection:** Iodine has been used for water disinfection in areas with limited access to clean drinking water. Research has shown that iodine can effectively kill waterborne pathogens and improve water quality.

6. Emergency Medicine:

- **Iodine for Wound and Skin Disinfection:** Iodine-based solutions are commonly used in emergency medicine to disinfect wounds and prepare patients for surgery or invasive procedures. Studies have demonstrated their effectiveness in reducing the risk of infection in emergency settings.

7. Viral Infections:

- **Iodine and Viral Infections:** Some research has explored the potential antiviral properties of iodine. While iodine is primarily known for its antibacterial properties, there is ongoing interest in understanding its effects on viruses, including influenza viruses and some enveloped viruses.

It's important to note that while iodine
has demonstrated antimicrobial
efficacy, its use should be in
accordance with established protocols
and guidelines. The concentration and
form of iodine, as well as the specific
microorganisms targeted, can
influence its effectiveness.
Additionally, consideration of
individual sensitivities and allergies is
essential when using iodine-based
products.

Numerous studies and scientific
investigations have confirmed the
antimicrobial properties of iodine,
making it a valuable tool in infection
control, wound care, and various
medical applications. Further research
continues to expand our
understanding of iodine's role in
combating microbial infections and its

potential applications in the healthcare field.

7.2 Iodine's Effects on Thyroid Disorders

Iodine plays a central role in thyroid function, and its availability can significantly impact thyroid health. Research has explored how iodine affects thyroid disorders, including its role in preventing thyroid dysfunction and its implications in managing thyroid-related conditions. Here, we delve into the effects of iodine on thyroid disorders:

1. Iodine Deficiency and Hypothyroidism:

- **Hypothyroidism** is a condition characterized by an underactive thyroid gland, leading to reduced production of thyroid hormones. Iodine deficiency is a well-established cause of hypothyroidism. When the body lacks sufficient iodine to produce thyroid hormones (T3 and T4), the thyroid gland can become enlarged (goiter) as it attempts to compensate for the deficiency.

2. Iodine Excess and Hyperthyroidism:

- **Hyperthyroidism** is the opposite of hypothyroidism and is characterized by an overactive thyroid gland, leading to excessive production of thyroid hormones. While iodine deficiency can lead to hypothyroidism, excessive iodine intake can also disrupt thyroid function and trigger or worsen hyperthyroidism, particularly in susceptible individuals.

3. Autoimmune Thyroid Diseases:

- **Hashimoto's Thyroiditis:** This autoimmune disease is characterized by inflammation and destruction of the thyroid gland. Some studies have suggested that excess iodine intake may contribute to the development or exacerbation of Hashimoto's thyroiditis in genetically susceptible individuals.

- **Graves' Disease:** Graves' disease is another autoimmune thyroid disorder characterized by an overactive thyroid. While the relationship between iodine and Graves' disease is complex, high iodine intake has been associated with an increased risk of developing Graves' disease in some populations.

4. Thyroid Nodules and Cancer:

- **Thyroid Nodules:** Iodine deficiency has been linked to the development of thyroid nodules, which are lumps or growths on the thyroid gland. While iodine supplementation may help reduce the size of certain benign thyroid nodules, its role in the management of nodules is still an area of research.

- **Thyroid Cancer:** Excessive iodine intake has been proposed as a potential risk factor for certain types of thyroid cancer, particularly in regions with high iodine intake. However, the relationship between iodine and thyroid cancer is complex and influenced by multiple factors.

5. Iodine and Thyroid Imaging:

- **Radiographic Contrast Media:** Iodine-based contrast agents are used in medical imaging procedures like CT scans and angiography to enhance the visibility of the thyroid and surrounding structures. While these agents provide valuable diagnostic information, they can temporarily affect thyroid function and may pose risks to individuals with preexisting thyroid disorders.

6. Thyroid Health Maintenance:

- **Balanced Iodine Intake:** Maintaining a balanced iodine intake is crucial for thyroid health. While iodine deficiency can lead to thyroid dysfunction, excessive iodine intake can have similar consequences. A balanced intake is essential for preventing both deficiency and excess.

Iodine plays a critical role in thyroid function and can have profound effects on thyroid disorders. Iodine deficiency can lead to hypothyroidism, while excessive iodine intake can disrupt thyroid function and contribute to hyperthyroidism or exacerbate autoimmune thyroid diseases. Achieving a balanced iodine intake tailored to individual needs is essential for supporting thyroid health and preventing thyroid-related disorders. Individuals with thyroid conditions should consult healthcare professionals for guidance on iodine intake and management of their specific thyroid disorder.

CHAPTER 8

Incorporating Iodine for Healing

Iodine-based products can be valuable tools in promoting healing and preventing infections in various healthcare settings. Proper use of these products and their integration into personal healthcare practices are essential for maximizing their benefits. Here's a guide on how to incorporate iodine for healing effectively:

8.1 Proper Use of Iodine-Based Products

a. Antiseptic Use:

- **Skin and Mucous Membrane Disinfection:** Iodine-based antiseptics like povidone-iodine are commonly used to disinfect the skin and mucous membranes before surgical procedures or the application of medical devices. Follow healthcare provider recommendations for the appropriate concentration and contact time.

- **Wound Care:** When using iodine-based solutions or dressings for wound care, clean the wound with a mild saline solution before applying iodine. Ensure that the wound is free of debris and foreign material. Follow healthcare provider instructions for dressing changes and the frequency of iodine application.

b. Topical Application:

- **Proper Concentration:** Iodine-based products are available in various concentrations. Choose the appropriate concentration based on the intended use and follow product instructions. Higher concentrations are generally used for surgical skin preparation, while lower concentrations may be suitable for minor wounds.

- **Avoid Excessive Application:** Do not overapply iodine-based products, as excessive iodine can lead to skin irritation or adverse effects. Apply a thin layer to the affected area or as directed by healthcare providers.

c. Safety Considerations:

- **Allergies and Sensitivities:** Be aware of iodine allergies or sensitivities, and inform healthcare providers if you have a known iodine allergy. Alternative antiseptics or wound care products may be used in such cases.

- **Monitoring:** If you experience any adverse reactions, such as skin redness, itching, or swelling, discontinue the use of iodine-based products and seek medical advice.

8.2 Integrating Iodine into Personal Healthcare

a. Consult with Healthcare Providers:

- **Thyroid Disorders:** If you have a thyroid disorder or are taking thyroid medication, consult with an endocrinologist or healthcare provider before using iodine supplements or iodine-rich products. They can help you determine the appropriate iodine intake for your specific condition.

- **Wound Care:** For minor wounds or burns at home, consult with a healthcare professional or pharmacist for guidance on using iodine-based products safely and effectively.

b. Balanced Diet:

- **Dietary Iodine:** Maintain a balanced diet that includes iodine-rich foods like seafood, dairy products, and iodized salt. This can help ensure you receive an adequate but not excessive amount of iodine.

- **Supplementation:** Avoid self-administered iodine supplements unless prescribed by a healthcare provider. Over-the-counter iodine supplements can lead to excessive iodine intake and thyroid dysfunction.

c. Personal Hygiene:

- **Oral Health:** If using iodine-based mouthwashes or oral antiseptics, follow the instructions provided and consult with a dentist or oral healthcare provider for recommendations tailored to your oral health needs.

- **Skin Health:** When using iodine-based topical products for skin care, be attentive to your skin's response. If you experience irritation, consult a dermatologist for guidance on alternative products or skincare routines.

d. Awareness of Iodine Content:

- **Food Labels:** Read food labels to be aware of iodine content in processed foods, particularly if you have dietary restrictions or allergies.

e. Regular Check-Ups:

- **Thyroid Monitoring:** If you have a thyroid disorder, schedule regular check-ups with your healthcare provider to monitor thyroid function and adjust treatment if necessary.

Incorporating iodine for healing and maintaining overall health requires careful consideration of individual needs, adherence to healthcare provider guidance, and awareness of iodine sources and products.

Balancing iodine intake is essential to prevent both deficiency and excess, ensuring optimal healing and thyroid function.

www.ingramcontent.com/pod-product-compliance
Lightning Source LLC
Chambersburg PA
CBHW070818280726

48660CB00016B/2128